SELF-LOVE JOURNAL
ISBN Hardcover: 979-8-3482-2997-9
ISBN Paperback: 979-8-3482-3004-3

SELF-LOVE JOURNAL with 7-SHIFT PLANNER
ISBN Hardcover: 979-8-3482-3012-8
ISBN Paperback: 979-8-3482-3023-4

My Self-Love Notes
The Most Important Relationship Is the One You Have with Yourself
Self-Love Is a Daily Practice

"You Don't Find Love, You Create Love" Sharon Esther Lampert

My Self-Love Planner - 7 Shifts

5-9 A.M. Early Bird

9-12 P.M.

12-3 P.M.

3-6 P.M.

6-9 P.M.

9-12 P.M.

12-3 A.M. Night Owl

My Self-Love Notes
The Most Important Relationship Is the One You Have with Yourself
Self-Love Is a Daily Practice

"You Don't Find Love, You Create Love" Sharon Esther Lampert

My Self-Love Planner - 7 Shifts

5-9 A.M. **Early Bird**

9-12 P.M.

12-3 P.M.

3-6 P.M.

6-9 P.M.

9-12 P.M.

12-3 A.M. **Night Owl**

My Self-Love Notes
The Most Important Relationship Is the One You Have with Yourself
Self-Love Is a Daily Practice

"You Don't Find Love, You Create Love" Sharon Esther Lampert

My Self-Love Planner - 7 Shifts

5-9 A.M. Early Bird

9-12 P.M.

12-3 P.M.

3-6 P.M.

6-9 P.M.

9-12 P.M.

12-3 A.M. Night Owl

My Self-Love Notes
The Most Important Relationship Is the One You Have with Yourself
Self-Love Is a Daily Practice

"You Don't Find Love, You Create Love" Sharon Esther Lampert

My Self-Love Planner - 7 Shifts

5-9 A.M. Early Bird

9-12 P.M.

12-3 P.M.

3-6 P.M.

6-9 P.M.

9-12 P.M.

12-3 A.M. Night Owl

My Self-Love Notes
The Most Important Relationship Is the One You Have with Yourself
Self-Love Is a Daily Practice

"You Don't Find Love, You Create Love" Sharon Esther Lampert

My Self-Love Planner - 7 Shifts

5-9 A.M. Early Bird

9-12 P.M.

12-3 P.M.

3-6 P.M.

6-9 P.M.

9-12 P.M.

12-3 A.M. Night Owl

My Self-Love Notes
The Most Important Relationship Is the One You Have with Yourself
Self-Love Is a Daily Practice

"You Don't Find Love, You Create Love" Sharon Esther Lampert

My Self-Love Planner - 7 Shifts

5-9 A.M. Early Bird

9-12 P.M.

12-3 P.M.

3-6 P.M.

6-9 P.M.

9-12 P.M.

12-3 A.M. Night Owl

My Self-Love Notes
The Most Important Relationship Is the One You Have with Yourself
Self-Love Is a Daily Practice

"You Don't Find Love, You Create Love" Sharon Esther Lampert

My Self-Love Planner - 7 Shifts

5-9 A.M. Early Bird

9-12 P.M.

12-3 P.M.

3-6 P.M.

6-9 P.M.

9-12 P.M.

12-3 A.M. Night Owl

My Self-Love Notes
The Most Important Relationship Is the One You Have with Yourself
Self-Love Is a Daily Practice

"You Don't Find Love, You Create Love" Sharon Esther Lampert

My Self-Love Planner - 7 Shifts

5-9 A.M. **Early Bird**

9-12 P.M.

12-3 P.M.

3-6 P.M.

6-9 P.M.

9-12 P.M.

12-3 A.M. **Night Owl**

My Self-Love Notes
The Most Important Relationship Is the One You Have with Yourself
Self-Love Is a Daily Practice

"You Don't Find Love, You Create Love" Sharon Esther Lampert

My Self-Love Planner - 7 Shifts

5-9 A.M. Early Bird

9-12 P.M.

12-3 P.M.

3-6 P.M.

6-9 P.M.

9-12 P.M.

12-3 A.M. **Night Owl**

My Self-Love Notes
The Most Important Relationship Is the One You Have with Yourself
Self-Love Is a Daily Practice

"You Don't Find Love, You Create Love" Sharon Esther Lampert

My Self-Love Planner - 7 Shifts

5-9 A.M. Early Bird

9-12 P.M.

12-3 P.M.

3-6 P.M.

6-9 P.M.

9-12 P.M.

12-3 A.M. Night Owl

My Self-Love Notes
The Most Important Relationship Is the One You Have with Yourself
Self-Love Is a Daily Practice

"You Don't Find Love, You Create Love" Sharen Esther Lampert

My Self-Love Planner - 7 Shifts

5-9 A.M. Early Bird

9-12 P.M.

12-3 P.M.

3-6 P.M.

6-9 P.M.

9-12 P.M.

12-3 A.M. Night Owl

My Self-Love Notes
The Most Important Relationship Is the One You Have with Yourself
Self-Love Is a Daily Practice

"You Don't Find Love, You Create Love" Sharon Esther Lampert

My Self-Love Planner - 7 Shifts

5-9 A.M. Early Bird

9-12 P.M.

12-3 P.M.

3-6 P.M.

6-9 P.M.

9-12 P.M.

12-3 A.M. Night Owl

My Self-Love Notes
The Most Important Relationship Is the One You Have with Yourself
Self-Love Is a Daily Practice

"You Don't Find Love, You Create Love" Sharon Esther Lampert

My Self-Love Planner - 7 Shifts

5-9 A.M. Early Bird

9-12 P.M.

12-3 P.M.

3-6 P.M.

6-9 P.M.

9-12 P.M.

12-3 A.M. Night Owl

My Self-Love Notes
The Most Important Relationship Is the One You Have with Yourself
Self-Love Is a Daily Practice

"You Don't Find Love, You Create Love" Sharon Esther Lampert

My Self-Love Planner - 7 Shifts

5-9 A.M. **Early Bird**

9-12 P.M.

12-3 P.M.

3-6 P.M.

6-9 P.M.

9-12 P.M.

12-3 A.M. **Night Owl**

My Self-Love Notes
The Most Important Relationship Is the One You Have with Yourself
Self-Love Is a Daily Practice

"You Don't Find Love, You Create Love" Sharon Esther Lampert

My Self-Love Planner - 7 Shifts

5-9 A.M. **Early Bird**

9-12 P.M.

12-3 P.M.

3-6 P.M.

6-9 P.M.

9-12 P.M.

12-3 A.M. **Night Owl**

My Self-Love Notes
The Most Important Relationship Is the One You Have with Yourself
Self-Love Is a Daily Practice

"You Don't Find Love, You Create Love" Sharon Esther Lampert

My Self-Love Planner - 7 Shifts

5-9 A.M. Early Bird

9-12 P.M.

12-3 P.M.

3-6 P.M.

6-9 P.M.

9-12 P.M.

12-3 A.M. Night Owl

My Self-Love Notes
The Most Important Relationship Is the One You Have with Yourself
Self-Love Is a Daily Practice

"You Don't Find Love, You Create Love" Sharon Esther Lampert

My Self-Love Planner - 7 Shifts

5-9 A.M. **Early Bird**

9-12 P.M.

12-3 P.M.

3-6 P.M.

6-9 P.M.

9-12 P.M.

12-3 A.M. **Night Owl**

My Self-Love Notes
The Most Important Relationship Is the One You Have with Yourself
Self-Love Is a Daily Practice

"You Don't Find Love, You Create Love" Sharon Esther Lampert

My Self-Love Planner - 7 Shifts

5-9 A.M. Early Bird

9-12 P.M.

12-3 P.M.

3-6 P.M.

6-9 P.M.

9-12 P.M.

12-3 A.M. Night Owl

My Self-Love Notes
The Most Important Relationship Is the One You Have with Yourself
Self-Love Is a Daily Practice

"You Don't Find Love, You Create Love" Sharon Esther Lampert

My Self-Love Planner - 7 Shifts

5-9 A.M. **Early Bird**

9-12 P.M.

12-3 P.M.

3-6 P.M.

6-9 P.M.

9-12 P.M.

12-3 A.M. **Night Owl**

My Self-Love Notes
The Most Important Relationship Is the One You Have with Yourself
Self-Love Is a Daily Practice

"You Don't Find Love, You Create Love" Sharon Esther Lampert

My Self-Love Planner - 7 Shifts

5-9 A.M. **Early Bird**

9-12 P.M.

12-3 P.M.

3-6 P.M.

6-9 P.M.

9-12 P.M.

12-3 A.M. **Night Owl**

My Self-Love Notes
The Most Important Relationship Is the One You Have with Yourself
Self-Love Is a Daily Practice

"You Don't Find Love, You Create Love" Sharon Esther Lampert

My Self-Love Planner - 7 Shifts

5-9 A.M. **Early Bird**

9-12 P.M.

12-3 P.M.

3-6 P.M.

6-9 P.M.

9-12 P.M.

12-3 A.M. **Night Owl**

My Self-Love Notes
The Most Important Relationship Is the One You Have with Yourself
Self-Love Is a Daily Practice

"You Don't Find Love, You Create Love" Sharon Esther Lampert

My Self-Love Planner - 7 Shifts

5-9 A.M. **Early Bird**

9-12 P.M.

12-3 P.M.

3-6 P.M.

6-9 P.M.

9-12 P.M.

12-3 A.M. **Night Owl**

My Self-Love Notes
The Most Important Relationship Is the One You Have with Yourself
Self-Love Is a Daily Practice

"You Don't Find Love, You Create Love" Sharon Esther Lampert

My Self-Love Planner - 7 Shifts

5-9 A.M. **Early Bird**

9-12 P.M.

12-3 P.M.

3-6 P.M.

6-9 P.M.

9-12 P.M.

12-3 A.M. **Night Owl**

My Self-Love Notes
The Most Important Relationship Is the One You Have with Yourself
Self-Love Is a Daily Practice

"You Don't Find Love, You Create Love" Sharon Esther Lampert

My Self-Love Planner - 7 Shifts

5-9 A.M. **Early Bird**

9-12 P.M.

12-3 P.M.

3-6 P.M.

6-9 P.M.

9-12 P.M.

12-3 A.M. **Night Owl**

My Self-Love Notes
The Most Important Relationship Is the One You Have with Yourself
Self-Love Is a Daily Practice

"You Don't Find Love, You Create Love" Sharon Esther Lampert

My Self-Love Planner - 7 Shifts

5-9 A.M. **Early Bird**

9-12 P.M.

12-3 P.M.

3-6 P.M.

6-9 P.M.

9-12 P.M.

12-3 A.M. **Night Owl**

My Self-Love Notes
The Most Important Relationship Is the One You Have with Yourself
Self-Love Is a Daily Practice

"You Don't Find Love, You Create Love" Sharon Esther Lampert

My Self-Love Planner - 7 Shifts

5-9 A.M. Early Bird

9-12 P.M.

12-3 P.M.

3-6 P.M.

6-9 P.M.

9-12 P.M.

12-3 A.M. Night Owl

My Self-Love Notes
The Most Important Relationship Is the One You Have with Yourself
Self-Love Is a Daily Practice

"You Don't Find Love, You Create Love" Sharon Esther Lampert

My Self-Love Planner - 7 Shifts

5-9 A.M. Early Bird

9-12 P.M.

12-3 P.M.

3-6 P.M.

6-9 P.M.

9-12 P.M.

12-3 A.M. Night Owl

My Self-Love Notes
The Most Important Relationship Is the One You Have with Yourself
Self-Love Is a Daily Practice

"You Don't Find Love, You Create Love" Sharon Esther Lampert

My Self-Love Planner - 7 Shifts

5-9 A.M. Early Bird

9-12 P.M.

12-3 P.M.

3-6 P.M.

6-9 P.M.

9-12 P.M.

12-3 A.M. Night Owl

My Self-Love Notes
The Most Important Relationship Is the One You Have with Yourself
Self-Love Is a Daily Practice

"You Don't Find Love, You Create Love" Sharon Esther Lampert

My Self-Love Planner - 7 Shifts

5-9 A.M. Early Bird

9-12 P.M.

12-3 P.M.

3-6 P.M.

6-9 P.M.

9-12 P.M.

12-3 A.M. **Night Owl**

My Self-Love Notes
The Most Important Relationship Is the One You Have with Yourself
Self-Love Is a Daily Practice

"You Don't Find Love, You Create Love" Sharon Esther Lampert

www.ingramcontent.com/pod-product-compliance
Lightning Source LLC
LaVergne TN
LVHW070121080526
838201LV00095B/250